AF583215

INTRODUCTION

Thank you for downloading this fantastic guide—**"9 Simple Exercises That Cure Your Body Pain."**

This eBook is contained of 9 simple exercises that are based on the outcomes of 1000's of my clients and their results from their existing problems.

As you browse the internet, u can get thousand of exercises that you can see literally but you may not know which one to follow? Or not. Isnt it?

And also, I can see most of the people are not really getting recovered completely from mild to moderate joint ache problems that they are suffering with for a long duration.

As a matter of help,I am releasing this eBook with these few simple hand picked exercises and when you apply for your existing problem, you can be recovered almost 80% from most of your ill chronic ailments.

It works like a magic.

Just BELEIVE AND FOLLOW. If you have doubts and fear on your mind before you do these exercises, I sincerely request you please do not follow these exercises.

Because holding doubts and suspicion in the mind, these exercises will never gonna work out. Please do not waste your time and money that is my humble request.

Let's Get Started!

NECK PAIN

Requirement-Yoga mat/bed mattresses,timer,water bottle

Time duration: 15-20 minutes

Session – preferable early morning.

Repetitions – 2 sets for each exercise.

1)Arching

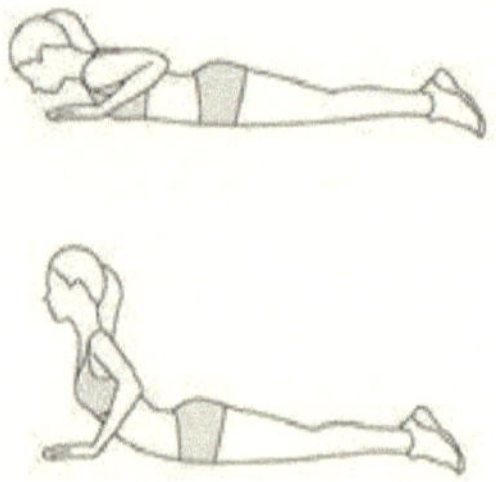

Step 1) - Lie on your tummy.

Step 2) - Keep your both hands next to your shoulders each.

Step 3) – Push your hands down in a downward pressure and arch your body like cobra and look up the ceiling.

Step 4) – Hold it for 30 counts

Note:Make sure your elbow is straight.If you cannot straighten your elbow due any arthritis or old aged,gradually try to straighten the elbow.

2)Head And Shoulder Lifting

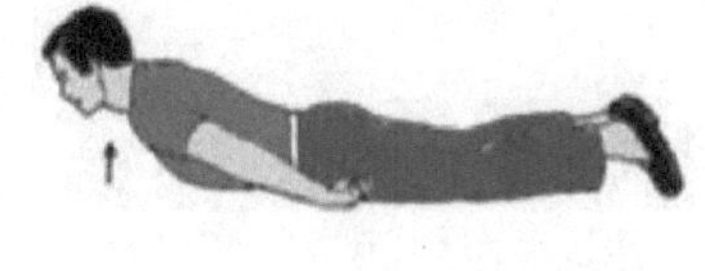

Step 1) – Lie on your tummy.

Step 2) – Keep your both arms sideways next to your body. Step 3) – Raise the head and both shoulders off the bed/floor

Step 4) – Keep your both arms either sideways or holding at the back.

Step 5) - Hold it for 30 counts.

3) Arm Backward Rotation

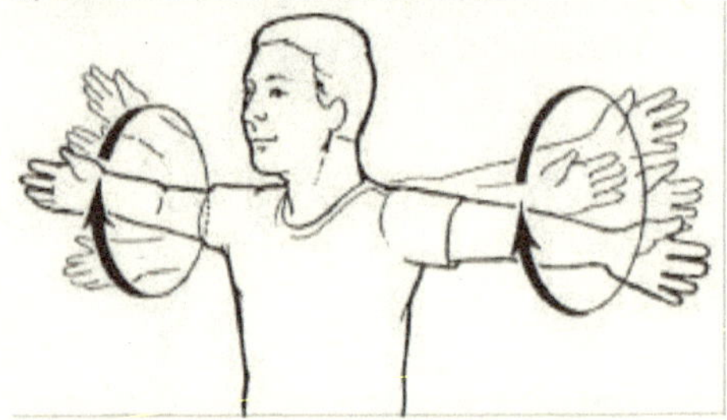

Step 1) – Touch your shoulders with your both hands with elbows bent.

Step 2) – Rotate arm in a backward/anti-clockwise direction.

Step 3) – Make sure the arm is moving from forward to backward direction(caution)

Step 4) – Repeat for 10 rotations.

4)Chest Open Up

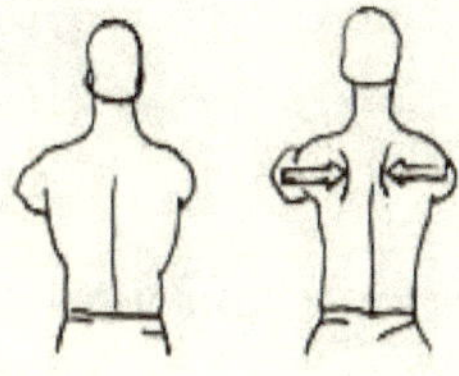

Step 1) – Keep your both arms in front of you and bent your elbows as shown in the pic.

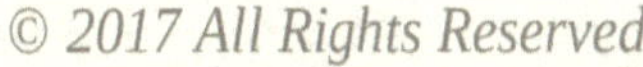

Step 2) – Open your chest by bringing your elbow in a backward direction.

Step 3) - Repeat for 10 rotations.

5)Chest Stretch

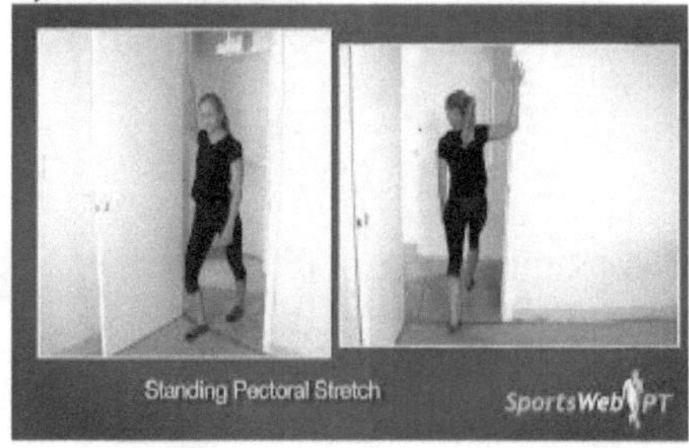

Step 1) – Stand straight next to wall as shown in the picture with elbows bent to 90.

Step 2) – Rest your other arm on your back.

Step 3) – Keep the same side leg forward(if you kept right arm on the wall,keep right leg forward)

Step 4) – Maintain the leg distance to the maximum but with in the limits.

Step 5) – Bend your front knee forward while fixing the elbow with the wall.

Step 6) – As you feel a stretch over the chest on the side where you kept your leg forward,hold it for 30 counts.

Step 7) – Repeat the stretch for other side as well.

6)Arm Stretch

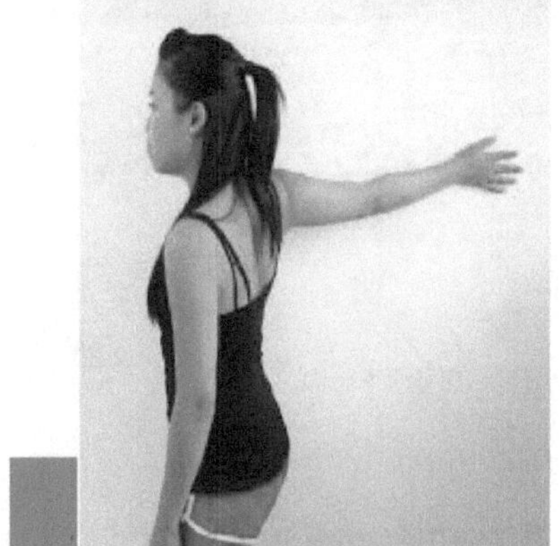

Step 1) – Stand straight next to wall as shown in the picture with elbows straight.

Step 2) – Rest your other arm on your back.

Step 3) – Keep your legs together with little gap in between.

Step 4) – Rotate your upper body to the opposite direction.

Step 5) – As you feel the stretch over the entire arm,hold it for 30 counts.

Step 6) – Repeat the stretch on other side as well.

Step 7) – Hold the stretch for 30 counts.

7)Neck-Shoulder Stretch

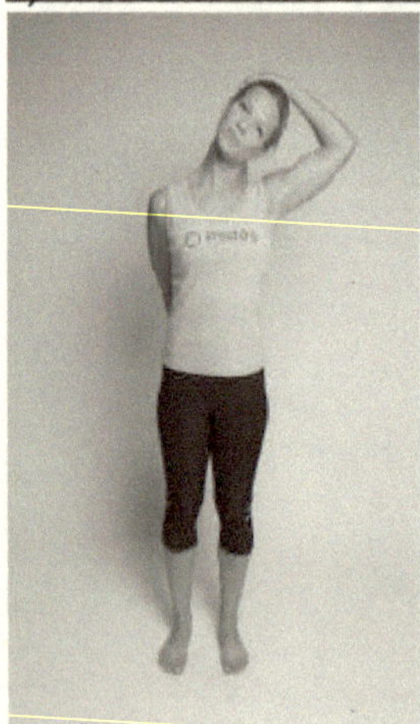

Step 1) – Lean your back on the wall as shown in the picture.

Step 2) – Lift one leg with knee bent and hold your thighs with your both hands.

Step 3) – Make sure your head and shoulders are touching the wall constantly.

Step 4) – Now hold the thighs with your both hands and push the thighs at a downward direction

Step 5) – You can feel the stretch from the neck to the shoulder part.

Step 6) – Repeat the same on the opposite side as well.

Step 7) – Hold the stretch for 30 counts.

8)Side Neck Stretch

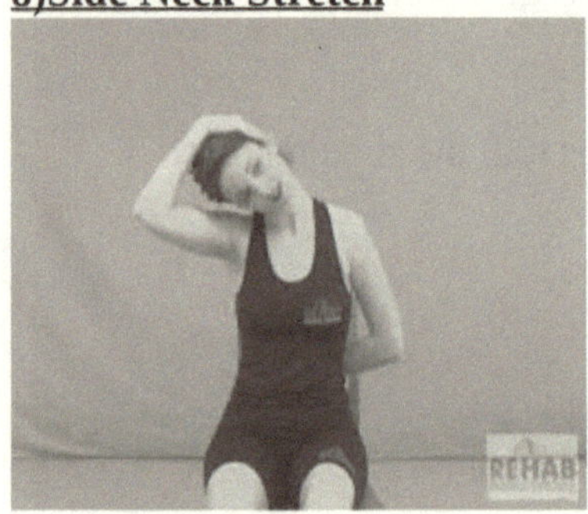

Step 1) – Sit/stand on the chair/bed.

Step 2) – Spine upright while holding one arm on the bed and the other arm on your opposite side of your head.

Step 3) – Pull the neck to the opposite direction while maintaining shoulder straight as shown in the picture.

Step 4) – You can feel a stretch exactly on the side of the neck.

Step 5) – Repeat the same on other side of the neck as well.

Step 6) – Hold stretches on each side for 30 counts.

10)Elbow Outward Rotation

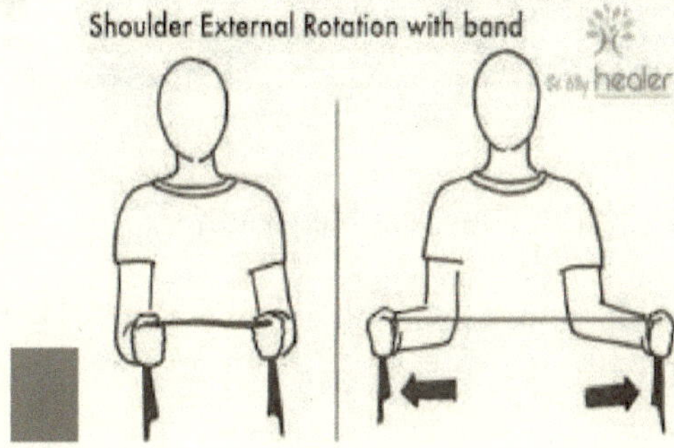
Shoulder External Rotation with band
healer

Step 1) – Stand straight with legs in line with your shoulder width.

Step 2) – Keep your arms sideways with elbows bent and hold dumbbells(1kg or 2kg) on both hands.

Step 3) – Make sure your elbow is touching the body and rotate the arm in an outward direction.

Step 4) – Hold for a sec and return back to neutral.

Step 5) – Do not touch both arms each other.

Step 6) – Repeat it for 10 repetitions.

<u>9)Arm Lifting On Tummy Position.</u>

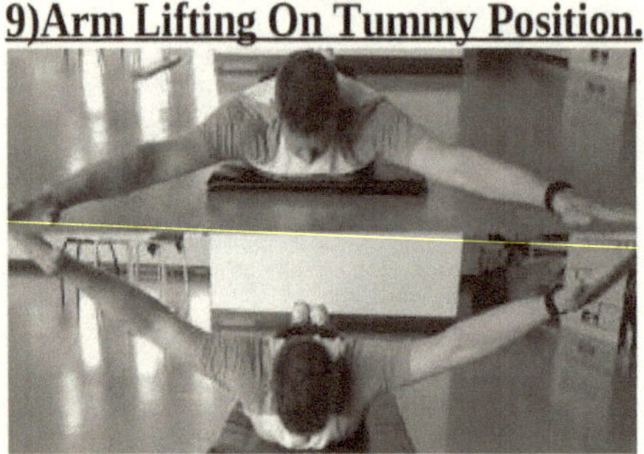

Step 1) – Lie down on your tummy on the floor.

Step 2) – Make sure your forehead is touching the floor.

Step 3) – Keep both arms sideways as shown in the picture i.e) 90 to your body.

Step 4) – Raise both arms off the floor and hold it for 30 counts.

Step 5) – You can feel a strength between the shoulder blades.

Step 6) – You can increase the counts even upto 50.

LOW BACK PAIN

1)Arching

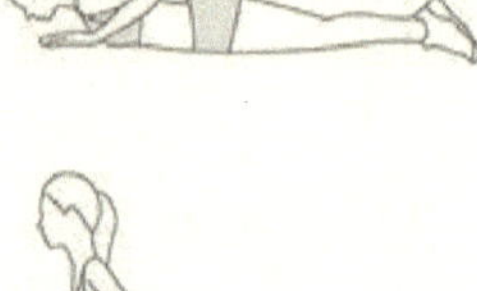

Step 1) - Lie on your tummy.

Step 2) - Keep your both hands next to your shoulders each.

Step 3) – Push your hands down in a downward pressure and arch your body like cobra and look up the ceiling.

Step 4) – Hold it for 30 counts

Note:Make sure your elbow is straight.If you cannot straighten your elbow due any arthritis or old aged,gradually try to straighten the elbow.

2)Head And Shoulder Lifting

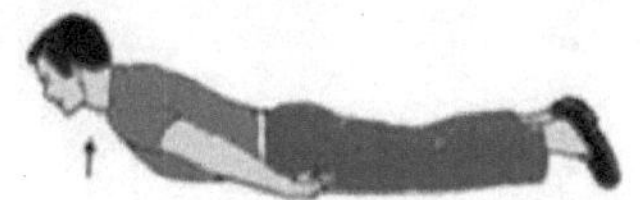

Step 1) – Lie on your tummy.

Step 2) – Keep your both arms sideways next to your body.

Step 3) – Raise the head and both shoulders off the bed/floor

Step 4) – Keep your both arms either sideways or holding at the back.

Step 5) - Hold it for 30 counts.

3)Hip Lifting

Bridging Exercise

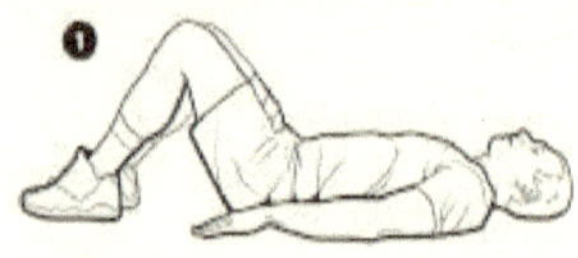

Lie flat on back with knees bent, feet planted flat on the floor.

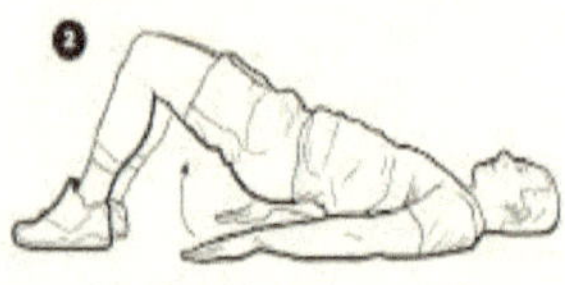

Tighten abdominal and buttock muscles and lift buttocks off the floor (repeat).

Step 1) – Lie on your back on the floor/yoga mat.

Step 2) – Keep your both arms sideways next to your body.

Step 3) – Bend both knees to 60 while feet touching the floor.

Step 4) – Slowly lift your hip as shown in the picture and hold it for 30 – 50 counts.

Step 5) – Make sure your hip,knee and chest all aligned in the same line.

4)Calf Stretch

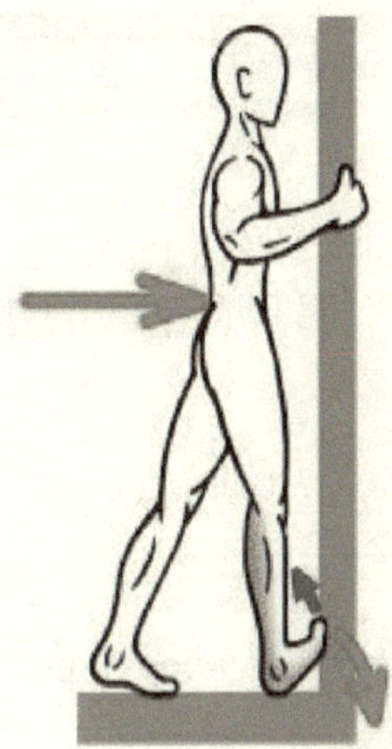

Step 1) – Stand straight in front of the wall with one leg forward with feet resting on the wall.

Step 2) – Make sure both knees are straight and arms touching the wall in a relaxed way.

Step 3) – Now slowly lift the heel of your back leg while feeling stretch over the calf of the front leg.

Step 4) – If you want more stretch,lift the heel more of your back leg.

Step 5) – Hold the stretch for 30 counts and repeat the stretch on other side as well.

5)Hamstring Stretch

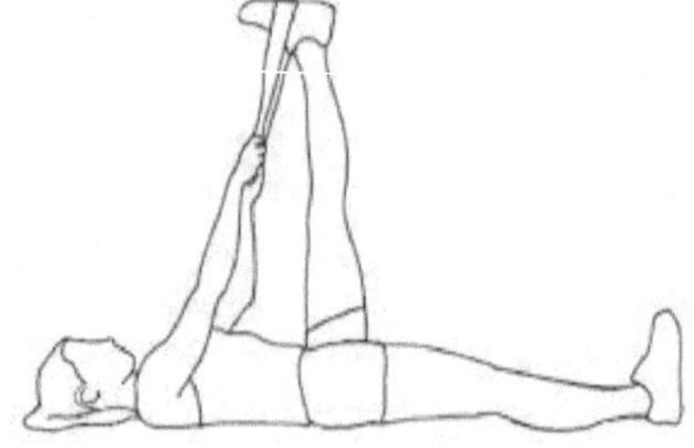

Step 1) – Stand straight while keeping one leg up on the chair/bed with knee straight.

Step 2) – Make sure your foot is pointing in the upward direction while the opposite leg looks straight

Step 3) – Now bend your body forward and try to touch the knee wit hyour both hands

Step 4) – Try to touch your toes and make it as a target and you can feel the strtech over the back thigh as you bend your body forward.

Step 5) – Hold the stretch for 30 counts and repeat the stretch on other side as well.

6)Front Thigh Stretch

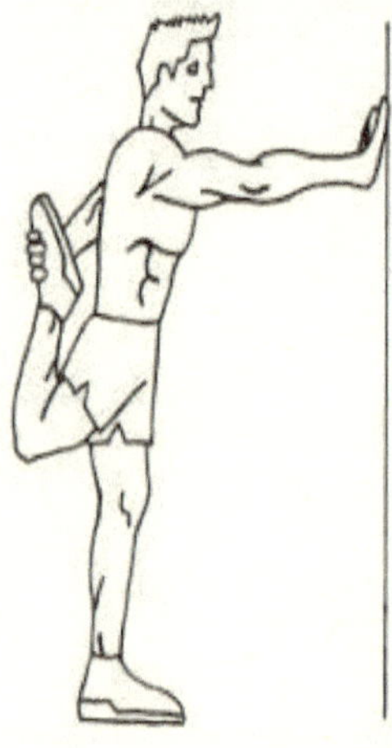

Step 1) – Stand straight in front of a wall and bend one knee while holding the ankle.

Step 2) – Keeping the body erect and pull the leg in a backward direction while look straight.

Step 3) – As you pull the leg back,you can feel a stretch over the front thigh.

Step 4) – Hold the stretch for 30 counts and repeat the stretch on the other side as well.

7)Butt Stretch

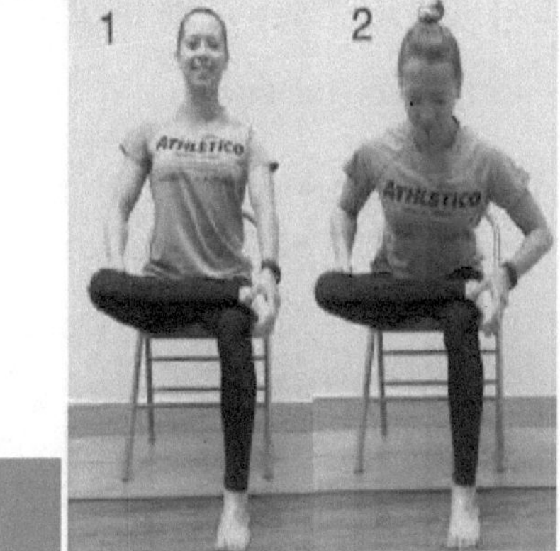

Step 1) – Sit on a chair/sofa with legs crossed as shown in the picture below.

Step 2) – Hold both arms together and keep it forward.

Step 3) – Now Bend your body forward as the other leg rests on the floor.

Step 4) – As you bend forward,you can feel a stretch on the butt.

Step 5) – Hold the stretch for 30 counts and repeat the stretch on other side as well.

8)Bird Dog Exercise

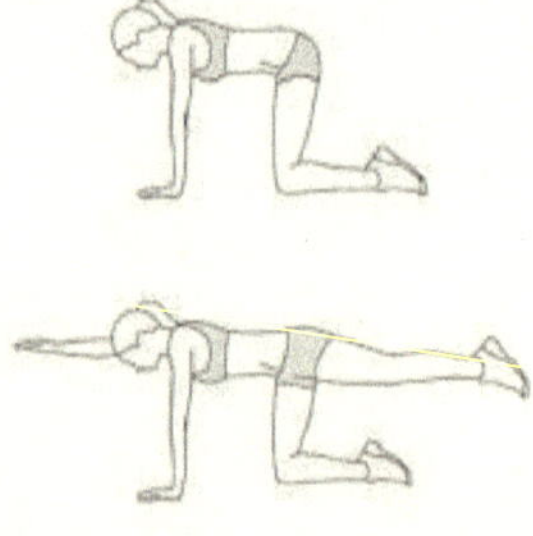

Step 1) – Kneel down on your legs and hands on the floor as shown in the picture .

Step 2) – Make sure the knees and hands falls on a straight line and it forms like a square.

Step 3) – Lift one arm and opposite leg simultaneously(for ex.while lifting left arm,lift your right leg and vice versa)

Step 4) – Make sure the elbows and knees are straight and face looks down.

Step 5) – Hold this position for 50 counts and repeat the same on the other side as well.

Caution:Not advised for old aged and knee arthritis persons.

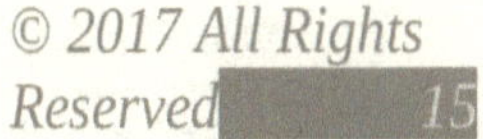

9)Plank

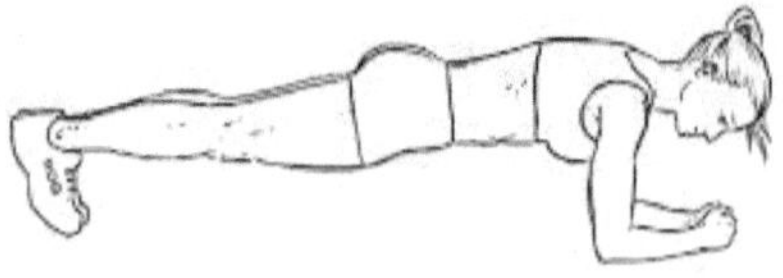

Step 1) – Lie on your tummy on the floor/yoga mat.

Step 2) – Place your forearms on the ground and make sure the elbow is aligned in line with the shoulders.

Step 3) – Clasp both hands together and rests your toes on the floor instead of whole ankle.

Step 4) – Push down your forearms and toes and lift the body and knees off the floor.

Step 5) – As you can see the whole body,butt and heel should be aligned in a straight line as like a wooden plank.

Step 6) – Hold this position as much as you can.Some people hold only for 10 counts whereas others hold for 2 minutes.But the the more time you hold ,more strength you will be gained.

Note :other exercises can be useful for low back such as Standing on one leg,Jogging,Jumping at one place or playing any sports.

SHOULDER PAIN

1)Pendular Exercises

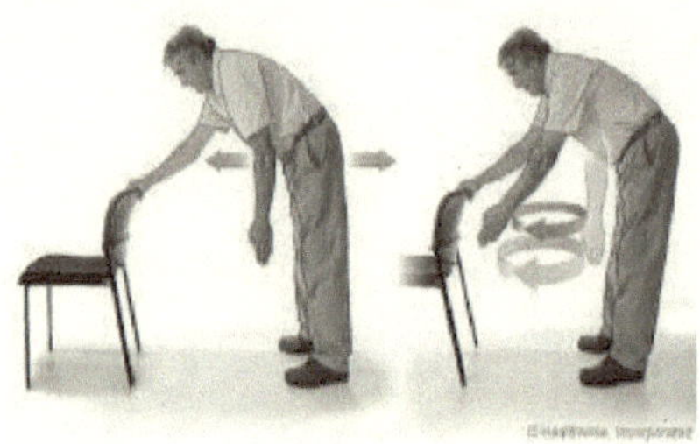

Step 1) – Stand next to a table/wall with body bent little forward as shown in the picture.

Step 2) – Place one hand on the table/wall while the other arm dangles down with a little weight that you can hold.

Step 3) – As you hold the weight,swing your arms forward and backward,sideways and rotate in both clockwise and anticlockwise direction.

Step 4) – You can do each movement for 10 repetitions.

Step 5) – Repeat the same on other side as well.

2)Shoulder Backward Rotation

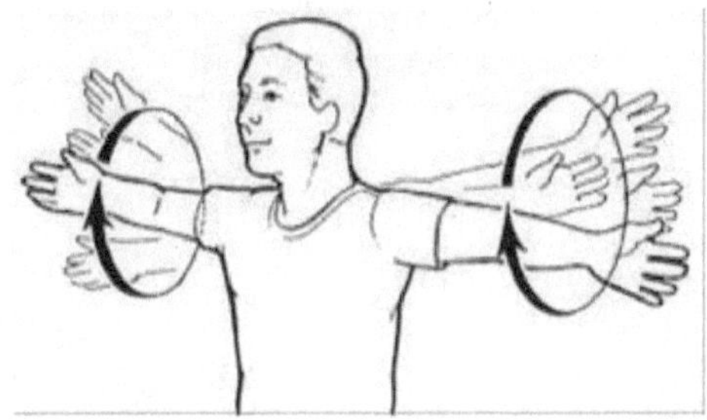

Step 1) – Touch your shoulders with your both hands with elbows bent.

Step 2) – Rotate arm in a backward/anti-clockwise direction.

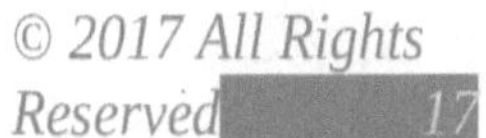

Step 3) – Make sure the arm is moving from forward to backward direction(caution)

Step 4) – Repeat for 10 rotations.

3)Chest Open Up

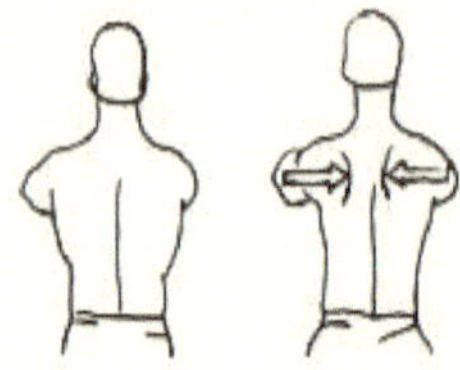

Step 1) – Keep your both arms in front of you and bent your elbows as shown in the pic.

Step 2) – Open your chest by bringing your elbow in a backward direction.

Step 3) - Repeat for 10 rotations.

4)Side Neck Stretch

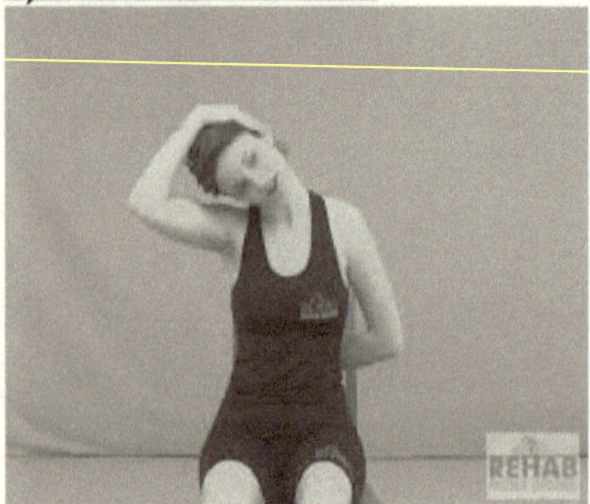

Step 1) – Sit on the chair/bed.

Step 2) – Spine upright while holding one arm on the bed and the other arm on your opposite side of your head.

Step 3) – Pull the neck to the opposite direction while maintaining shoulder straight as shown in the picture.

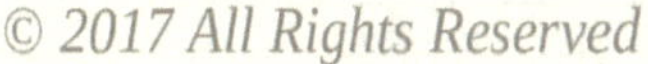

Step 4) – You can feel a stretch exactly on the side of the neck.

Step 5) – Repeat the same on other side of the neck as well.

Step 6) – Hold stretches on each side for 30 counts.

5)Elbow Outward Rotation

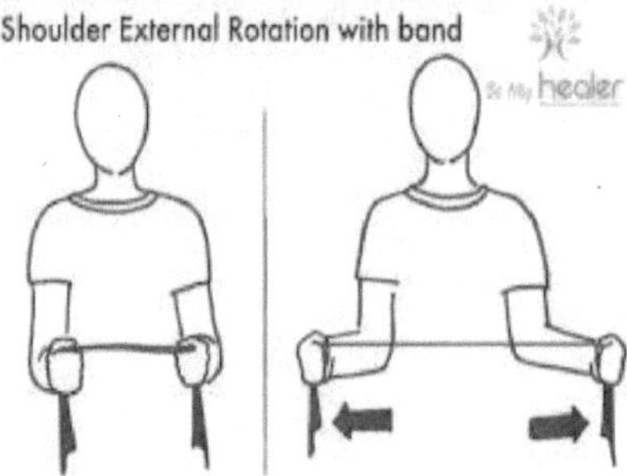

Step 1) – Stand straight with legs in line with your shoulder width.

Step 2) – Keep your arms sideways with elbows bent and hold dumbbells(1kg or 2kg) on both hands.

Step 3) – Make sure your elbow is touching the body and rotate the arm in an outward direction.

Step 4) – Hold for a sec and return back to neutral.

Step 5) – Do not touch both arms each other.

Step 6) – Repeat it for 10 repetitions.

6)Chest Stretch

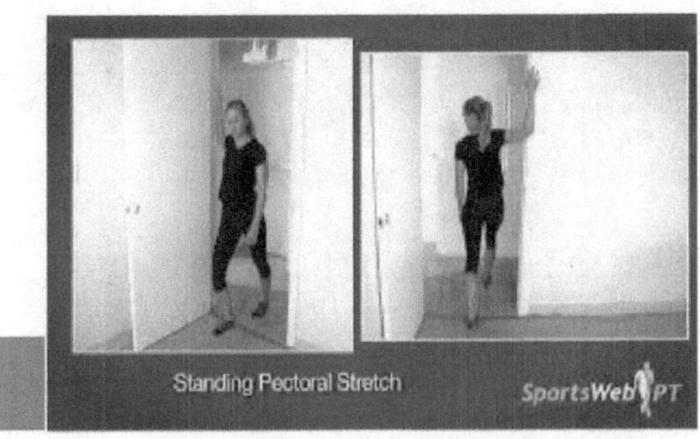
Standing Pectoral Stretch
SportsWeb PT

Step 1) – Stand straight next to wall as shown in the picture with elbows bent to 90.

Step 2) – Rest your other arm on your back.

Step 3) – Keep the same side leg forward(if you kept right arm on the wall,keep right leg forward)

Step 4) – Maintain the leg distance to the maximum but with in the limits.

Step 5) – Bend your front knee forward while fixing the elbow with the wall.

Step 6) – As you feel a stretch over the chest on the side where you kept your leg forward,hold it for 30 counts.

Step 7) – Repeat the stretch for other side as well.

7)Arm Stretch

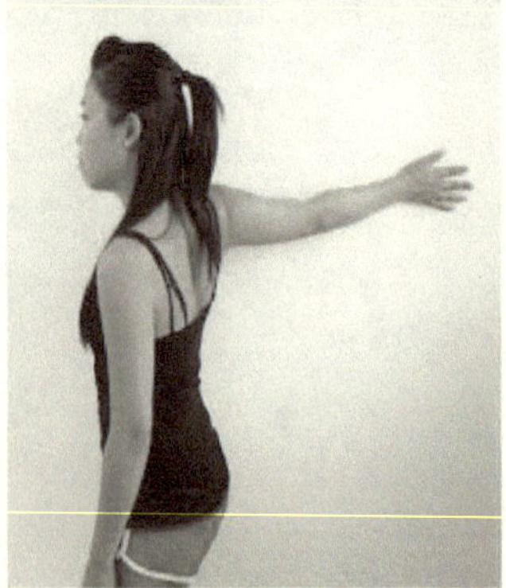

Step 1) – Stand straight next to wall as shown in the picture with elbows straight.

Step 2) – Rest your other arm on your back.

Step 3) – Keep your legs together with little gap in between.

Step 4) – Rotate your upper body to the opposite direction.

Step 5) – As you feel the stretch over the entire arm,hold it for 30 counts.

Step 6) – Repeat the stretch on other side as well.

Step 7) – Hold the stretch for 30 counts.

8)Neck-Shoulder Stretch

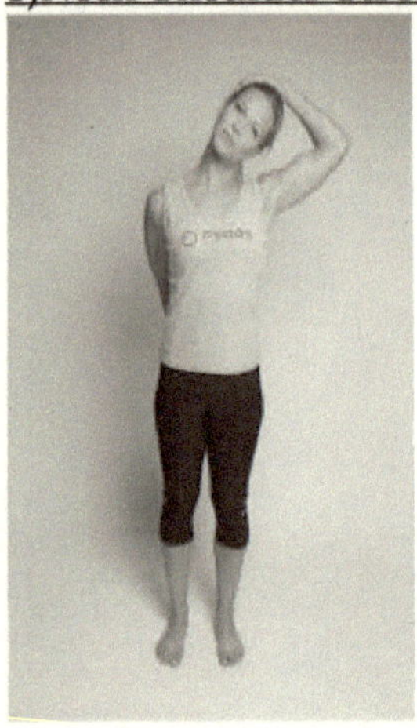

Step 1) – Lean your back on the wall as shown in the picture.

Step 2) – Lift one leg with knee bent and hold your thighs with your both hands.

Step 3) – Make sure your head and shoulders are touching the wall constantly.

Step 4) – Now hold the thighs with your both hands and push the thighs at a downward direction

Step 5) – You can feel the stretch from the neck to the shoulder part.

Step 6) – Repeat the same on the opposite side as well.

Step 7) – Hold the stretch for 30 counts.

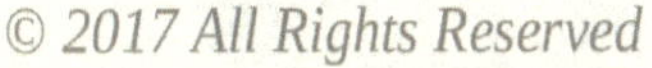

9)Fit Band Exercises

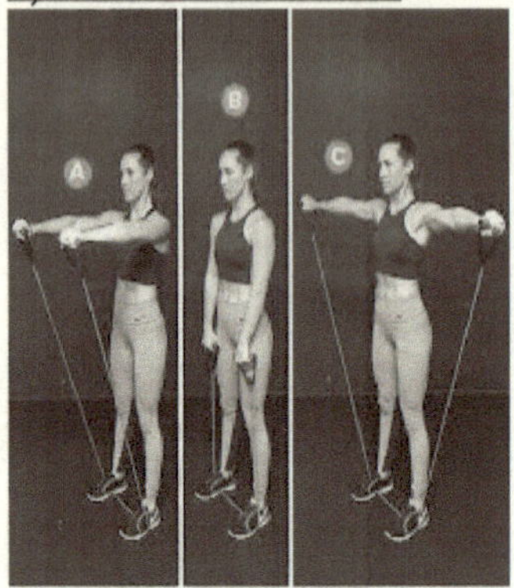

Fit band is a resistance band or elastic band that is used to strengthen the muscles all parts of the busy particularly for shoulder,knees,elbows and ankles. As such,fit band strengthens all groups of shoulder muscles:front,back and sideways.

Step 1) – Stand straight on your shoulder width.

Step 2) – Hold one end of the band with one hand whereas the other end down the foot as shown in the picture.

Step 3) – Place other arm on your back and lift the arm in a sideward direction while pulling the band sideways.

Step 4) – Repeat the same in a forward and backward direction as well.

Step 5) – Repetitions – 10 for each direction.

Note : As fit band is a very effective exercise for strength training but should be used in a proper manner.

The best way to do fit band is in 1:2 ratio i.e) 1 second up movement 2 second down movement that means as you move your arms in an upward direction,move at a speed rate of 2 seconds while coming down at a rate of 1 second speed.

in short,going up is fast,coming down is slow. Exercise no 5 can also be done with this band.

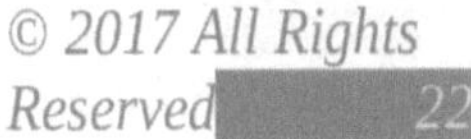

KNEE PAIN

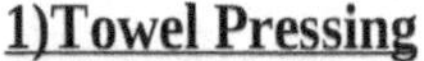

1)Towel Pressing

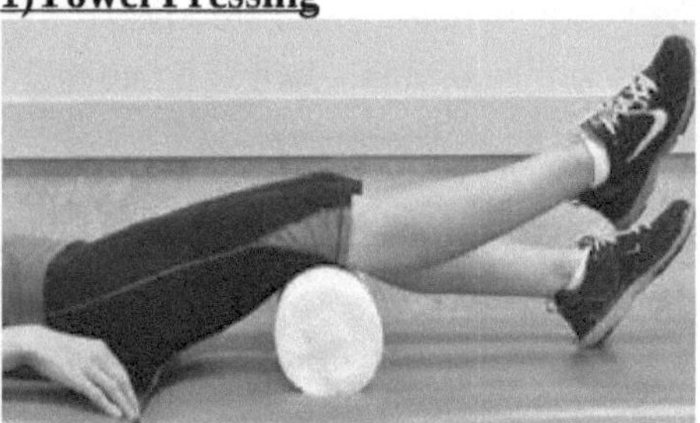

Step 1) – Sit on the floor/yoga mat with legs straight

Step 2) – Place one towel under the knee and press the towel down while foot comes up.

Step 3) – Hold the press for 30 – 50 counts.

Step 4) – Repeat the same on the other leg as well.

2)Leg Lifting

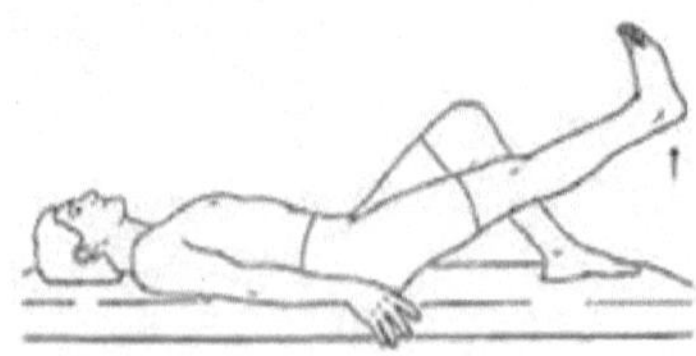

Step 1) – Lie down flat on the floor/yoga mat.

Step 2) – Lift one leg with slight knee bent s shown in the picture Step 3) – Hold the leg for 30 – 50 counts.

Step 4) – Repeat the same on the other leg as well.

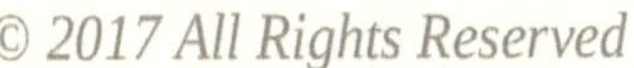

3)Calf Stretch

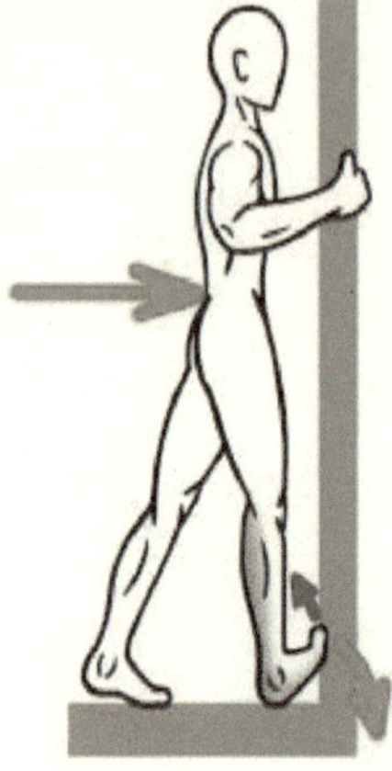

Step 1) – Stand straight in front of the wall with one leg forward with feet resting on the wall.

Step 2) – Make sure both knees are straight and arms touching the wall in a relaxed way.

Step 3) – Now slowly lift the heel of your back leg while feeling stretch over the calf of the front leg.

Step 4) – If you want more stretch,lift the heel more of your back leg.

Step 5) – Hold the stretch for 30 counts and repeat the stretch on other side as well.

4)Hamstring Stretch

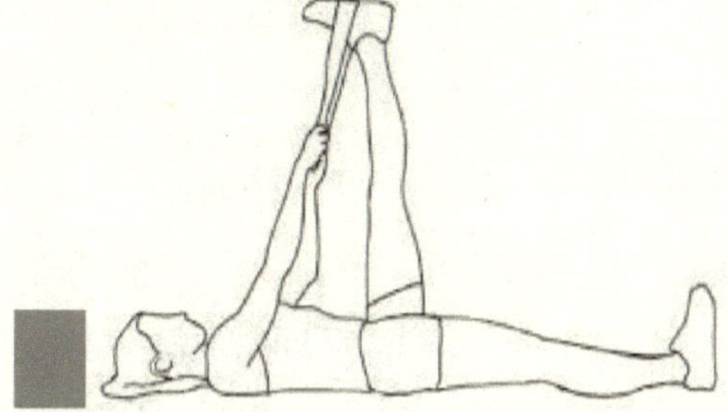

Step 1) – Stand straight while keeping one leg up on the chair/bed with knee straight.

Step 2) – Make sure your foot is pointing in the upward direction while the opposite leg looks straight

Step 3) – Now bend your body forward and try to touch the knee with your both hands

Step 4) – Try to touch your toes and make it as a target and you can feel the stretch over the back thigh as you bend your body forward.

Step 5) – Hold the stretch for 30 counts and repeat the stretch on other side as well.

5)Front Thigh Stretch

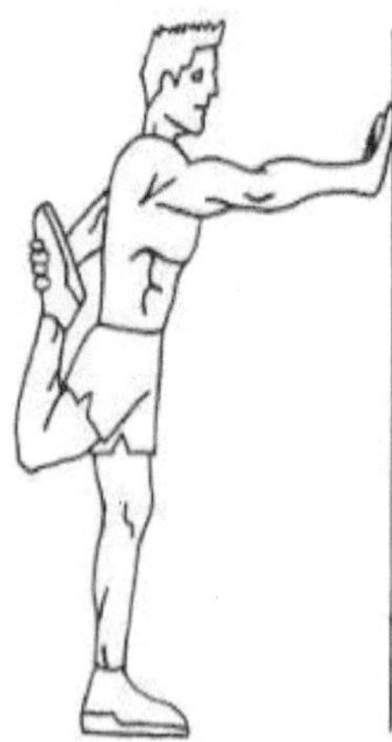

Step 1) – Stand straight in front of a wall and bend one knee while holding the ankle.

Step 2) – Keeping the body erect and pull the leg in a backward direction while look straight.

Step 3) – As you pull the leg back,you can feel a stretch over the front thigh.

Step 4) – Hold the stretch for 30 counts and repeat the stretch on the other side as well.

6)Squats

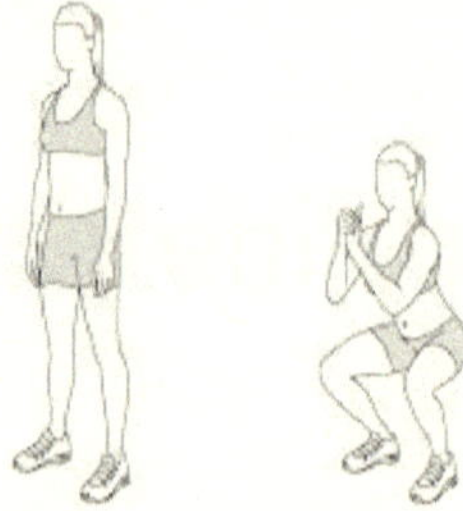

As squats are the very effective strength training for your knee and it is useful for any aged people.

Step 1) – Stand straight on your shoulder width.

Step 2) – Arms forward and bend the knee slowly while lowering the hip and back down.

Step 3) – Make sure the knees are not ahead of the toe line as shown in the picture.

Step 4) – Hold the position for 30-50counts.

Note : As I see many clients are doing squats by bringing the knee in front of the toe line since its the wrong method,I would not advise you to follow.

Progressively,you can strength your knee further by doing squats with weights like this below one.

7)Knee Straightening

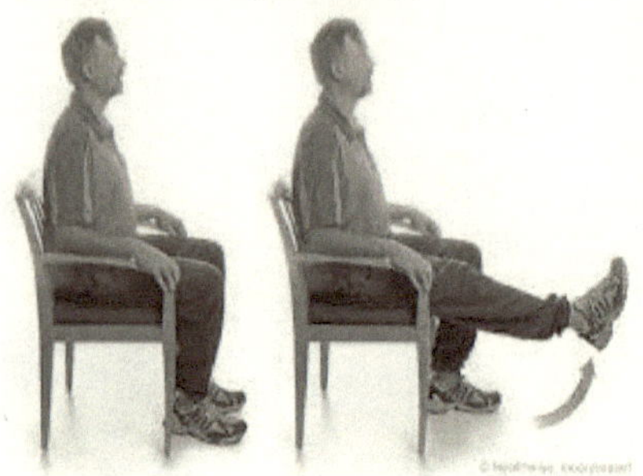

Step 1) – Sit Straight on a chair/sofa with feet resting on the ground.

Step 2) – keeping the body erect.arms sideways,slowly lift one leg and straight the knee.

Step 3) – Foot is straight and the toes are pointing upwards.

Step 4) – Hold this position for 30-50counts.

As this exercise is very effective for old aged.

And also,you can do this exercise at the fitness clubs either by machines or fit bands.

8)Knee Pressing

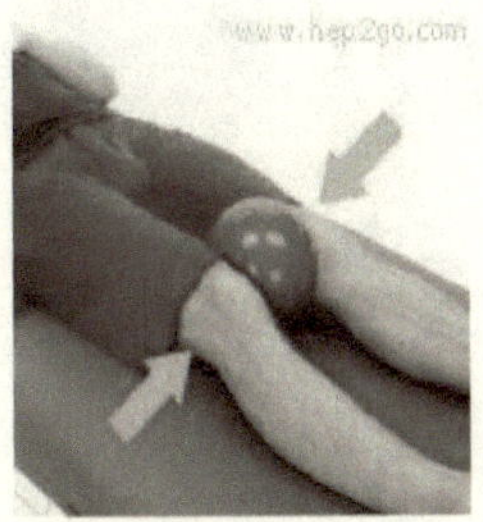

Step 1) – Sit on the floor/mat with knees straight.

Step 2) – Place a towel between the knee and press the towel with your knees and hold.

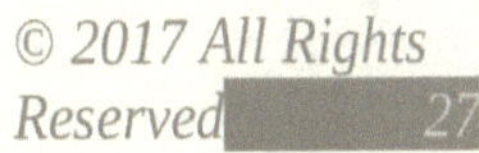

Step 3) – Foot is relaxed and normal

Step 4) – Hold the press for 30-50counts.

9)Knee Curl

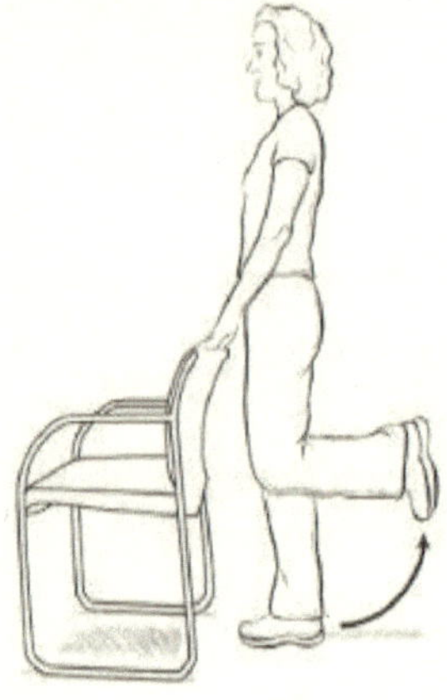

Step 1) – Stand straight in front of the wall as shown in the picture.

Step 2) – Intermittently,bend and straighten one knee in a gradual way.

Step 3) – Follow the 1:2 ratio,as you bend move fast at 1 sec speed rate and when you straight the knee,move slowly at 2 sec speed rate

Step 4) – Hold the press for 30-50counts.

As we have covered the major parts of the body such as spine,shoulder and knee,the rest of the body parts like elbow,ankle and fingers do not have specific set of exercises.

If in case of muscle or bone related pain,just follow these exercises for the initial 2-3 days,you can see the guaranteed results of 20-30% pain relief.As such,continue for a week or so,you will be out of your problem to almost 70%.

If in case the pain doesn't reduce even 10% despite doing the exercises for almost a week please consult with your physician doctor/specialist.

In my experience,nearly 1000's of my clients got nearly 80% pain relief by just following these above mentioned basic exercises.

Pay Attention

As the rule of this book i.e) 9 simple exercises for the joint pain,I would list down 3 exercises for some case diagnosis.

Note:Please do all 9 exercises but concentrate more on these 3 exercises particularly.

Cervical problem – Neck pain exercises(2,3,5)

Peri arthritis shoulder – Shoulder exercises (2,6,7)

Lumbar problem – Low back pain (1,3,4)

Knee arthritis(OA,RA) – Knee pain (1,3,4)

www.ingramcontent.com/pod-product-compliance
Lightning Source LLC
LaVergne TN
LVHW041254150826
845673LV00008B/2585

* 9 7 9 8 5 3 8 9 8 2 9 7 4 *